KIDNEY FRIENDLY FOOD LIST

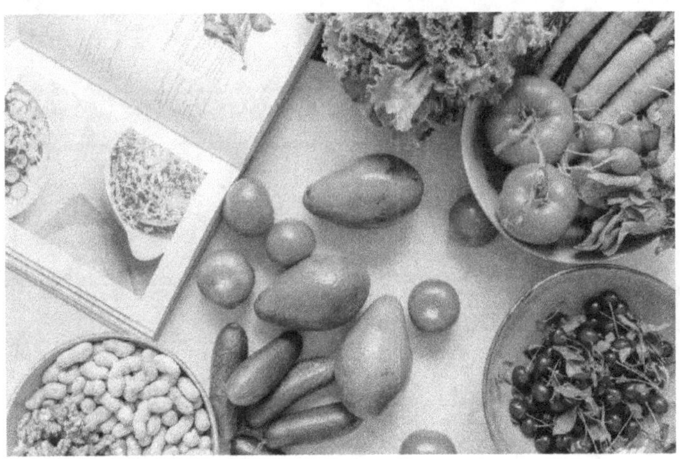

Low Sodium, Low Potassium Foods and Nutritional Guidance for Managing Kidney Disease

BELL QUINTANA

TABLE OF CONTENT

INTRODUCTION

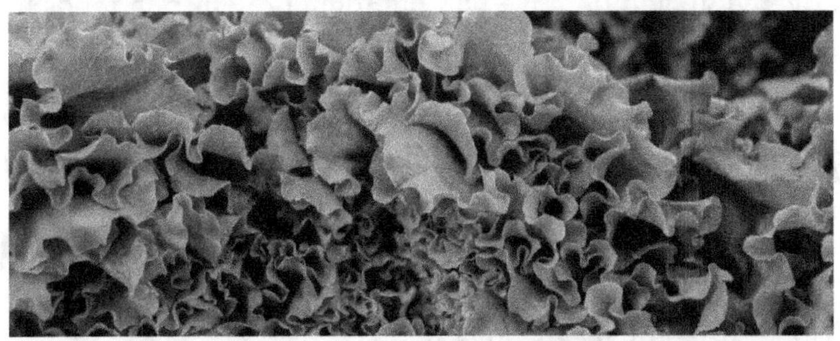

Welcome to the "Kidney Friendly Food List"! If you've picked up this book, you're most likely looking for information on how to nourish your kidneys and improve your overall health. You've come exactly to the right place!

In this book, we will go on a journey to discover the amazing world of kidney-friendly eating habits. Whether you're dealing with kidney issues, trying to prevent them, or simply want to understand more about how your food affects your overall health, this book will help you every step of the way.

So, what can you expect from the next pages? Let me give you a taste!

First, we'll cover the principles of kidney-friendly nutrition. We'll look at the relevance of important nutrients and how they affect kidney function. You'll learn about portion control and how to navigate the shopping aisles like a professional.

Next, prepare for the ultimate kidney-friendly food list! From low-potassium powerhouses to low-phosphorus gemstones and sodium-savvy options, we've got you covered. In addition, we will highlight protein-rich foods to keep you satisfied and energized.

But that is not all! We'll provide nutritional facts and serving size recommendations to assist you make informed decisions. Then we'll roll up our sleeves and get down to the business of meal planning. With sample meal plans and clever tactics, you'll be able to prepare delicious and kidney-friendly meals quickly.

Cooking enthusiasts rejoice! Our chapter on cooking for kidney health is jam-packed with insights and strategies to help you create delicious kidney-friendly meals. Say goodbye to dull and hello to delectable meals that promote your health.

But we won't stop there. Oh no! We'll look at the broader panorama of lifestyle factors that affect kidney health, including the significance of exercise, stress management, and quality sleep.

Let's not forget about hydration. We'll look at the critical link between hydration and kidney function and provide you with recommendations for maintaining appropriate fluid balance.

Throughout the book, you'll find helpful insights to help you on your path.

So, grab a cozy spot, settle in, and get ready to nourish your kidneys and promote your well-being. With "Kidney Friendly Food List" as your trusted companion, you'll be well on the way to a healthier and happier you!

Now let's go on this amazing adventure together. Here's a little glimpse at what's in store...

Understanding Kidney Health

Our kidneys are unsung heroes, working tirelessly behind the scenes to remove waste and extra fluids from our blood while maintaining a delicate balance that keeps our systems functioning properly. To begin a journey toward kidney-friendly nutrition, it is critical to grasp the fundamentals of kidney function.

Picture your kidneys as a master chemists, conducting a symphony of filtration and regulation. They not only eliminate waste but also help to maintain an appropriate electrolyte and fluid balance. When this symphony is disrupted, it can cause a variety of health problems, emphasizing the significance of preventative kidney care.

Understanding how these essential organs work lays the groundwork for making informed food choices that promote and maximize their performance.

CHAPTER 1

Fundamentals of Kidney-Friendly Eating

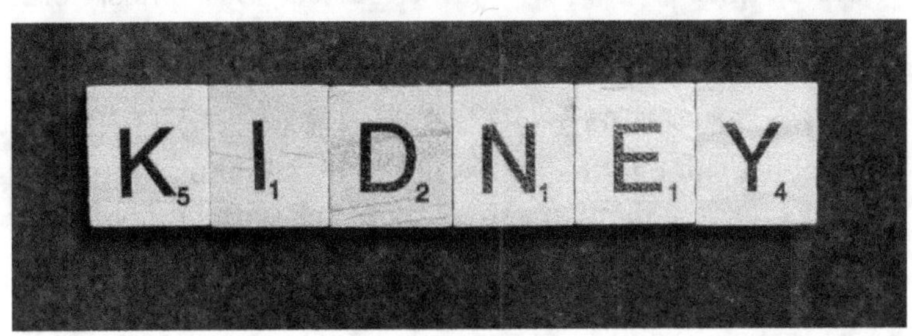

Understanding the principles of kidney-friendly food is similar to memorizing the notes before performing a symphony. We're about to start on a journey in which your taste buds and kidneys will become best friends. So let's get to the heart of the matter.

Key Nutrients and Their Effects on Kidney Health

Consider your kidneys to be the conductors of a large symphony, with the nutrients in your food serving as the players playing various instruments. Too much of one, not enough of another, and you end up with a cacophony rather than a symphony. Let's get to know our nutrient superstars and divas: potassium, phosphorus, sodium, and protein.

Potassium: This MVP is necessary for heart and muscle function, but excessive amounts might strain your kidneys. Fear not, we'll walk you through a slew of low-potassium options that will keep your heart humming without overwhelming your kidneys.

Phosphorus: Phosphorus, like the bass player, is often found in places that are not expected. Low-phosphorus gems allow your kidneys to function properly.

Sodium: The subtle cause of the bloated feeling. We'll unravel the salt enigma and look at low-sodium alternatives that will make your taste receptors dance without disrupting your kidney rhythm.

Protein: The building block of muscles and tissues, yet too much can be a burden on your kidneys. Fear not, we'll introduce you to protein-rich options that will keep your muscles in top shape without straining your kidneys.

Let the nutrient music start!

CHAPTER 2

Kidney-Friendly Food Guide

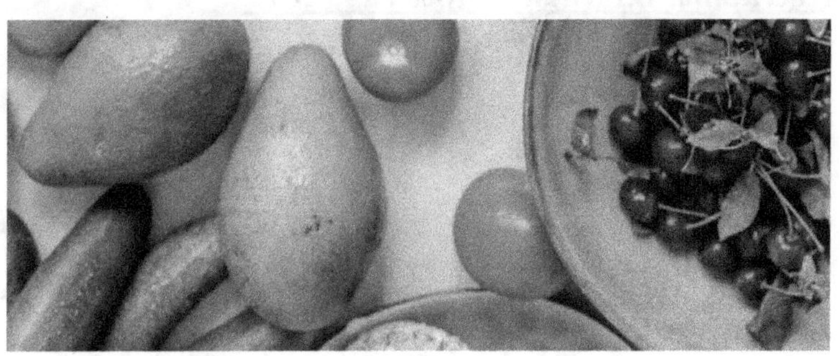

In this chapter, we reveal the pinnacle of kidney-friendly eating: the ultimate food list designed to improve your kidney health. Prepare to discover a treasure trove of delicious and nourishing options that will make your taste buds sing and your kidneys thrive. From low-potassium powerhouses to low-phosphorus gems and sodium-conscious options, we've compiled a complete list to help you create meals that are both delicious and nutritious. So, grab your shopping list and get ready to discover the culinary delights that await you in the world of kidney-friendly foods!

Low Potassium Foods

Welcome to the world of low potassium treats! Managing potassium intake is critical for kidney health, and we've compiled a list of delectable meals that won't raise your potassium levels. Let's delve into these kidney-friendly options, complete with nutritional information and serving size guidelines to keep your nutrient intake in check.

1) Cucumber:

Nutritional Information (per cup, sliced):

- Potassium (147 mg)
- Phosphorus (24 mg)
- Sodium: 2 mg.
- Protein: 0.6g -

Serving size Recommendation: Enjoy as a refreshing snack or mix into salads in 1/2 cup portions.

2. Strawberries:

Nutritional Information (per cup, whole):

- Potassium (233 mg)
- Phosphorus (24 mg)
- Sodium: 1 mg.
- Protein: 1 g.

Serving Size Recommendation: Enjoy a cup of fresh strawberries as a delicious and kidney-friendly dessert.

3. Bell peppers (red or green):

Nutritional Information (per medium-sized pepper):

- Potassium: 210 mg -
- Phosphorus: 18 mg -
- Sodium: 3 mg
- Protein: 1 g -

Serving size Recommendation: Add to stir-fries or serve as a crunchy snack in moderation.

4. Cauliflower:

Nutritional Information (per cup, chopped):

- Potassium (176 mg)
- Phosphorus, 44 mg
- Sodium: 30 mg.
- Protein: 2 grams.

Serving Size: Recommendation: Use as a low-potassium replacement for mashed potatoes in half a cup portions.

5. Pineapple:

Nutritional Information (per cup, chunks):

- Potassium: 180 mg.
- Phosphorus (13 mg)

- Sodium: 1 mg.
- Protein: 1 g.

<u>Serving Size: Recommendation:</u> Add a tropical flavor to your diet with 1/2 cup of fresh pineapple.

6. Berries (blueberries or raspberries):

<u>Nutritional Information (per cup):</u>

- Potassium: 114-144 mg (varies by berry)
- Phosphorus (22 mg)
- Sodium: 1 mg.
- Protein: 1-2 g (varies per berry)

<u>Serving size recommendation:</u> Sprinkle 1/4 cup over yogurt or cereal.

7. Onions:

<u>Nutritional Information (for a medium-sized onion)</u>

- Potassium (210 mg)
- Phosphorus: 38 mg.
- Sodium: 4 mg.
- Protein: 2 grams.

<u>Serving Size: Recommendation:</u> To add flavor to your recipes, include 1/2 cup sautéed onions.

Incorporate these low-potassium items into your everyday diet while keeping portion amounts in mind. With these delectable options, you can eat a kidney-friendly diet without sacrificing taste or diversity.

Low Phosphorus Foods*

Now, let's look at low-phosphorus miracles, the unsung heroes of kidney-friendly diets. Balancing phosphorus consumption is critical for kidney health, and we've compiled a list of delicious alternatives that won't tip the scales. Prepare to appreciate these nutrient-dense dishes, along with nutritional information and serving size suggestions to keep your phosphorus levels under control.

1. Egg whites:

Nutritional Information (per large egg white):

- Phosphorus: 5 mg -
- Potassium: 55 mg -
- Sodium: 55 mg
- Protein: 3.6 g -

Serving Recommendation: Whip up a phosphorus-friendly omelet with 2-3 egg whites.

2. Skinless Chicken Breast:

Nutritional Information (per 3-ounce cooked portion):

- Phosphorus, 180 mg
- Potassium: 256 mg.
- Sodium: 74 mg.
- Protein: 27 grams.

Serving size recommendation: A 3-ounce portion offers a protein boost that is phosphorus-controlled.

3. White Bread (Enriched):

Nutritional Information (per slice):

- Phosphorus (30 mg)
- Potassium (18 mg)
- Sodium: 80 mg.
- Protein: 2 grams.

Serving Size Recommendation: Use in moderation, with 1-2 slices per sandwich or toast.

4. White rice (cooked):

Nutritional values (per cup):

- Phosphorus: 68 mg.
- Potassium (35 mg)
- Sodium: 1 mg.
- Protein: 4 g.

Serving size recommendation: For a kidney-friendly starch, add 1/2 to 1 cup to your meals.

5. Apples:

Nutritional Information (Medium-Sized Apple)

- Phosphorus (10 mg)
- Potassium (195 mg)
- Sodium: 0 mg.
- Protein: 0.5 grams.

Serving Size: Recommendation: For a low-phosphorus snack, try a medium-sized apple.

6. Green beans (fresh):

Nutritional Information (per cup, cooked):

- Phosphorus (36 mg)
- Potassium (211 mg)
- Sodium: 1 mg.
- Protein: 2 grams.

Serving Size Recommendation: Include in meals with 1/2 to 1 cup servings.

7. Peaches (canned with juice and drained):

Nutritional Information (per cup):

- Phosphorus: 28 mg

- Potassium: 232 mg -
- Sodium: 0 mg
- Protein: 1 g

<u>Serving size Recommendation:</u> Eat in moderation, using 1/2 cup servings.

Incorporate these low-phosphorus items into your diet while paying attention to portion quantities. With these nutrient-dense selections, you can create a kidney-friendly diet that is both tasty and healthy.

Low Sodium Options

Ah, the desire of flavor without excessive sodium intake! In this part, we'll explore the world of low-sodium miracles to keep your kidneys satisfied and your taste buds happy. From savory to sweet, we've identified options that let you enjoy every bite without the sodium. Let's take a look at these palate-pleasing options, packed with nutritional information and serving size suggestions to ensure a great balance.

1. Salmon (fresh):

<u>Nutritional Information (per 3-ounce cooked portion):</u>

- Sodium: 50 mg.
- Potassium (370 mg)
- Phosphorus (213 mg)
- Protein: 22 grams.

Serving Size: Recommendation: With a 3-ounce serving, you can get a heart-healthy protein boost while being low in sodium.

2. Quinoa:

Nutritional data (per cup, cooked):

Sodium: 13 mg.
Potassium (318 mg)
Phosphorus (281 mg)
Protein: 8 grams.

Serving Size: Recommendation: Use 1/2 to 1 cup servings in meals for a low-sodium grain choice.

3. Greek Yogurt (Unsweetened)

Nutritional data (per 6-ounce container):

- Sodium: 60 mg,
- potassium: 240 mg
- phosphorus: 200 mg
- Protein: 15 grams.

Serving Size: Recommendation: 6-ounce portions make an excellent low-sodium snack or breakfast option.

4. Bell peppers (yellow or orange):

Nutritional Information (per medium-sized pepper):

- Sodium: 3 mg.
- Potassium: 256 mg.
- Phosphorus (18 mg)
- Protein: 1 g

Serving size Recommendation: Use sparingly in recipes or as a crunchy snack.

5. Oats (steel-cut, unsalted):**

Nutritional Information (per cup, cooked):

- Sodium: 2 mg.
- Potassium: 148 mg
- phosphorus: 77 mg.
- Protein: 5 grams.

Serving Size: Recommendation: Start your day with 1/2 to 1 cup of low-sodium oatmeal.

6. Cherries (fresh):

Nutritional Information (per cup):

- Sodium: 0 mg.
- Potassium (306 mg)

- Phosphorus (18 mg)
- Protein: 1 gram.

<u>Serving Size: Recommendation:</u> Serve as a sweet, low-sodium snack in 1/2 cup portions.

7. Broccoli:

<u>Nutritional Information (per cup, cooked):</u>

- Sodium: 30 mg.
- Potassium, 457 mg
- Phosphorus (50 mg)
- Protein: 3 grams.

<u>Serving Size:</u> Recommendation: Incorporate this low-sodium cruciferous vegetable into your meals in 1/2 to 1 cup servings.

With these low-sodium selections, you may enjoy the richness of your meals while keeping sodium under control. Experiment with these delectable options, modifying the portion amounts to meet your dietary requirements and taste preferences.

CHAPTER 3

Nutritional Information and Serving Size

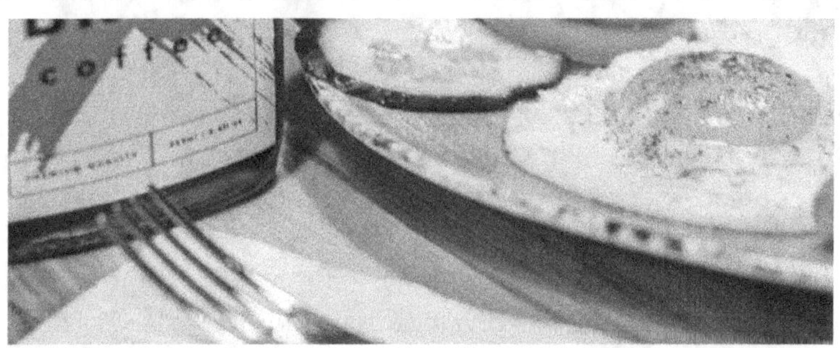

Welcome to the backstage tour of your meals, where we'll break down the nutritional value and perfect the art of portion control. Consider this chapter your own compass, guiding you through the complex terrain of nutrients and ensuring you strike all the proper notes with portion amounts. Let's get into the specifics, harmonizing flavor and function to create a nutritional symphony.

Understanding Nutritional Labels

Nutritional labels can be confusing with so many numbers and percentages, but don't worry! With some direction, you'll be able to navigate them like a seasoned explorer. Let's go on a trip to decode these labels and understand the key components that influence kidney health.

Potassium is a critical mineral that supports muscular function, neuronal communication, and fluid homeostasis. However, for people with reduced renal function, controlling potassium intake is critical. Scan the label for potassium concentration, and choose items with lower potassium levels to maintain a kidney-friendly diet. Keep a watch out for phrases like "potassium chloride" and "potassium bicarbonate," which indicate potassium additives.

Phosphorus: Ah, phosphorus – the stealthy ninja of the nutrient world. Phosphorus, which is often found in processed foods and additives, can have a negative impact on kidney health if consumed excessively. Check the label for phosphorus content, emphasizing whole, unprocessed foods and avoiding phosphorus additions if feasible. Remember that components such as "phosphate" or "phosphoric acid" indicate the existence of phosphorus additions.

SODIUM:

Sodium, a flavor enhancer we love to hate. While sodium is required for many body activities, excessive sodium consumption can cause high blood pressure and kidney strain. Check the label for salt content, and choose low-sodium or sodium-free products whenever possible. Be aware of hidden sodium in packaged foods, sauces, and condiments, and opt for fresh, whole foods wherever feasible.

Protein is essential for muscle and tissue development and must be included in every diet. However, for people with renal problems, managing protein intake is critical to preventing excessive load on the kidneys. Pay attention to the protein content on the label, and aim for a balance that fits your dietary requirements without overburdening your kidneys. To preserve kidney health, eat lean protein sources such as poultry, fish, tofu, and lentils and limit your portion sizes.

By becoming familiar with these crucial features on nutritional labels, you will be able to make more informed decisions that benefit your kidney health. Remember to prioritize whole, unprocessed foods and follow labels to create a kidney-friendly diet that feeds both body and soul.

Ideal Serving Sizes for Optimal Kidney Health

Portion control: Let's decipher the mysteries of serving sizes so your plate is a masterpiece, not a mountain. Here is a snapshot:

1. Proteins:
- **Chicken or Fish:** 3 ounces (equivalent to a deck of cards) for a protein-rich, kidney-friendly meal.
- **Eggs:** Use 1-2 eggs for a filling and nutrient-dense portion.

2. Grains:
- **Quinoa or rice:** 1/2 to 1 cup is an ideal amount for a substantial but kidney-friendly side dish.

3. Dairy:

- **Greek Yogurt:** 6 oz - a creamy and protein-rich dish without exceeding your phosphorus limit.
- **Cottage Cheese:** 1/2 cup - a nice protein boost without the extra sodium.

4. Fruits:

- **Berries:** 1/4 to 1/2 cup provides a blast of sweetness without the potassium excess.

5. Vegetables:

- **Leafy Greens:** Unlimited - fill your plate with these low-phosphorus, low-potassium gems.

6. Snack:

- **Nuts:** 1 ounce is a crunchy and kidney-friendly food when portioned correctly.

With this nutritional understanding and quantity control, you can create a dish that not only satisfies your taste buds but also nurtures your kidneys. So, let's confidently navigate the culinary seas, creating meals that are both delicious and kidney-friendly.

CHAPTER 4

Meal Plan Strategies

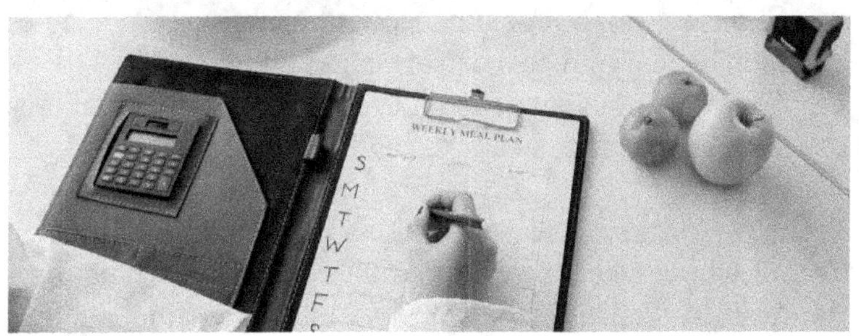

Meal planning is your secret weapon for achieving kidney-friendly joy! In this chapter, we'll look at how to prepare meals that not only taste good but also nourish your kidneys. Prepare to create a symphony of tastes with our balanced and kidney-friendly meal solutions. Furthermore, we provide sample meal plans suited to varied dietary requirements, guaranteeing that there is something delicious for everyone at the table.

Building Balanced and Kidney-Friendly Meals

Creating meals that work well with your kidneys is an art, and we're going to become meal maestros. Let us break it down:

1. Protein: Consume lean protein sources such as chicken, fish, tofu, and lentils.

- Choose serving proportions that deliver a protein boost without overwhelming your kidneys.
- For a full and well-balanced meal, combine proteins with nutritious grains or vegetables.

2. The Veggie Variety: Enjoy a variety of bright vegetables - the more the merrier!
- Choose low-potassium, low-phosphorus vegetables such as leafy greens, carrots, and bell peppers.
- To keep things interesting, use varied cooking methods such as roasting, steaming, and sautéing.

3. Carb Control: Choose whole grains like quinoa, brown rice, or whole wheat pasta for a nutrient-dense carb option.
- Maintain a healthy balance by keeping portion amounts in check.

4. Fruit Finesse:
- Consume fruits in moderation, opting for low-potassium alternatives like berries or apples.
- Fruits can be used as natural sweeteners or to make pleasant side dishes.

5. Savvy Seasonings:
- Use kidney-friendly herbs and spices.
- Use less salt and explore with tasty alternatives such as garlic, lemon, or vinegar.

6. Hydration Highlights: Stay hydrated!
- Water is your closest buddy; strive for at least 8 cups each day.

Sample Meal Plans for Different Dietary Needs

\At this point, let's put theory into practice with some tantalizing sample meal plans designed to suit various dietary needs.

1. Low-Potassium Symphony:

Breakfast: Scrambled eggs with spinach and a side of sliced peaches.
For Lunch: Grilled chicken salad with cucumber, cherry tomatoes, and a vinaigrette dressing.
Dinner: Your Baked salmon with quinoa & steamed green beans.

2. Low-Sodium Delight:

Breakfast: Greek yogurt parfait with low-sodium granola and berries.
For Lunch: Turkey and avocado wrap with a side of carrot sticks.
For Dinner: Your Shrimp stir-fry with snap peas & quinoa.

3. Low-Phosphorus Feast:

Breakfast: Oatmeal with sliced strawberries.
Lunch: Lentil soup with a side of mixed greens.
Dinner: Your Stir-fried tofu with broccoli & brown rice.

4.   Protein Powerhouse:

Breakfast: Smoothie with protein powder, almond milk and banana.
Lunch: Quinoa bowl with grilled chicken, black beans, and salsa.
For Dinner: Baked cod with sweet potato wedges and asparagus.

Feel free to mix and match, tailoring these regimens to your tastes and nutritional needs. With these methods and example menus in your culinary arsenal, you'll be well on your way to creating meals that not only benefit your kidney health but also rekindle your enjoyment for great and nutritious foods!

CHAPTER 5

Cooking for Kidney Health

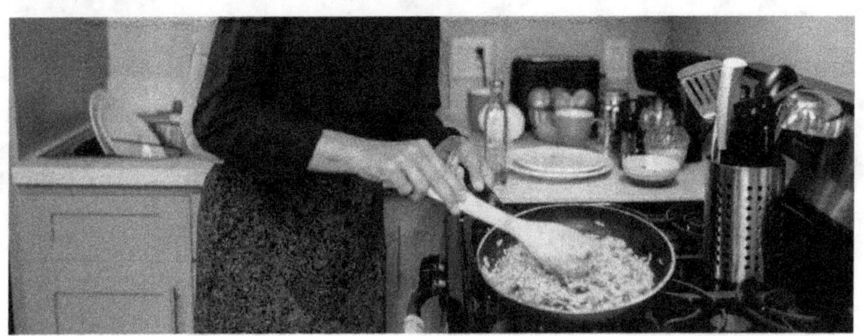

Cooking becomes a culinary canvas when you paint with kidney-friendly strokes! In this chapter, we put on our chef hats to investigate cooking methods that reduce potassium, phosphorus, and sodium. Plus, we've got some brilliant ingredient alternatives under our sleeves, since who says kidney-friendly can't be delicious?

Cooking Techniques to Reduce Potassium, Phosphorus, and Sodium

1. The Water Soak Ballet:
- Soaking lowers potassium and phosphorus levels, making these protein powerhouses more kidney-friendly.
- Say goodbye to extra sodium with a thorough rinse after the soak.

2. The Double Potassium Twist: Boiling and draining are effective methods for controlling potassium levels in vegetables.
- To dramatically lower potassium content, boil your potassium-rich vegetables and then discard the water.
-

3. The Phosphorus Paso Doble: Use cooking procedures that remove phosphorus.
- Techniques such as boiling, blanching, and soaking can help you fight phosphorous.

4. The Sodium Shuffle: Replace sodium with fresh herbs, spices, and lemon for added taste.
- For a low-sodium culinary tango, skip the salt during cooking and instead experiment with post-cooking seasoning.

1. 5. The Baking Ballet: Baking is a low-maintenance dance for both sweet and savory delights.
- Enhance flavors without adding unnecessary sodium, and let your oven do the work for a hassle-free, kidney-friendly performance.

Smart ingredient substitutions

1. Replace salt with herbs or spices such as basil, thyme, cumin, or paprika to reduce sodium intake. Enhance your food with delectable alternatives that won't raise your sodium levels.

2. Sweet Potatoes vs. White Potatoes: Switch from potassium-rich white potatoes to kidney-friendly sweet potatoes. Get your comfortable potato fix with consuming less potassium.

3. Phosphorus-Free Grains: Switch to whole grains like quinoa or bulgur for a phosphorus-free option. Improve your grain game without jeopardizing kidney health.

4. Dairy Distinction: Low-Phosphorus Options: Choose low-phosphate dairy or non-dairy alternatives. Enjoy the creaminess without the excessive phosphorous content.

5. Sodium Sleight of Hand: Use vinegar-based dressings instead of high sodium sauces. Enjoy the tanginess without the sodium hangover.

Embrass these culinary techniques and ingredient replacements as your kitchen companions, resulting in masterpieces that celebrate both flavor and kidney health. It's time to move through your culinary masterpieces with a rhythm that is both excellent for your taste buds and your kidneys!

CHAPTER 6

Beyond the Plate—Lifestyle and Kidney Health

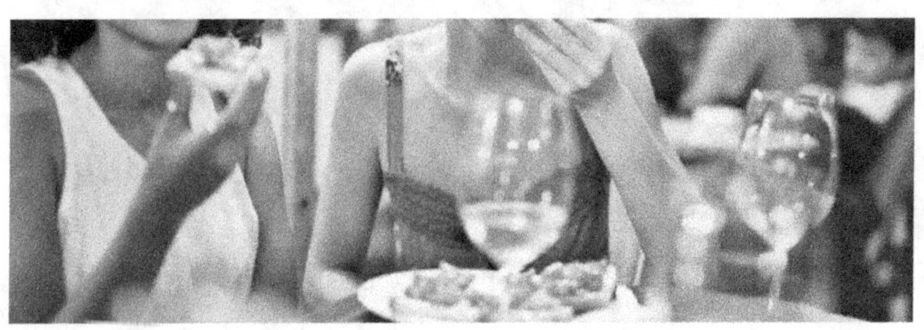

In this chapter, we'll go beyond the plate and into the realms of lifestyle, because holistic health is more than just what you eat. Prepare to dance to the beat of wellness as we explore the dance of exercise, the soothing melody of stress management, and the lullaby of quality sleep - all of which contribute to your kidney's health.

How Exercise Affects Kidney Health

1. Cardio Cha-Cha: Cardiovascular exercise is a heart-pumping dance that your kidneys love.

- Exercise like brisk walking, jogging, or cycling to improve blood flow and renal function.

- Aim for at least 150 minutes of moderate-intensity activity each week; your kidneys will give you a standing ovation.

2. Strength Tango: Focus on strength training as a partner dance for muscle growth.
- Gaining muscular mass can help you maintain a healthy weight and improve renal function.
- Include resistance exercises 2-3 times each week for a strong routine that keeps your kidneys in great form.

Stress Management and its Impact on Kidneys

1. Meditation Waltz: Stress can have a significant impact on kidney health.
- Incorporate mindfulness practices such as meditation to alleviate stress and create a peaceful mental environment.
- A few minutes of meditation per day can lead to a stress-free kidney zone.

2. Yoga Serenade: Enjoy a relaxing yoga session for your body and mind.
- Yoga not only relieves stress, but it also develops flexibility and balance, providing a comprehensive approach to kidney health.
- Practice your favorite yoga positions while listening to calming self-care music.

Importance of Quality Sleep for Kidney Function

1. Slumber Sonata:
- Sleep is essential for general health and kidney function.
- Aim for 7-9 hours of excellent sleep per night to help your body, particularly your kidneys, renew and heal.
- Establish a nighttime routine, dim the lights, and let the sleep sonata to soothe you into a sound sleep.

2. Technology Tango:
- Make sure you turn off screens at least one hour before bedtime.
- Blue light emitted by screens can disrupt your sleep symphony; instead, choose a technological tango that encourages improved sleep quality.

As we conclude our kidney-friendly trip, remember that a healthy lifestyle includes more than just what you eat. Accept the dance of exercise, sway to the beat of stress management, and let the soothing symphony of quality sleep be the perfect complement to your kidney-friendly lifestyle. Your kidneys are not only survivors; they are the stars of this fitness show!

CHAPTER 7

Stay Hydrated

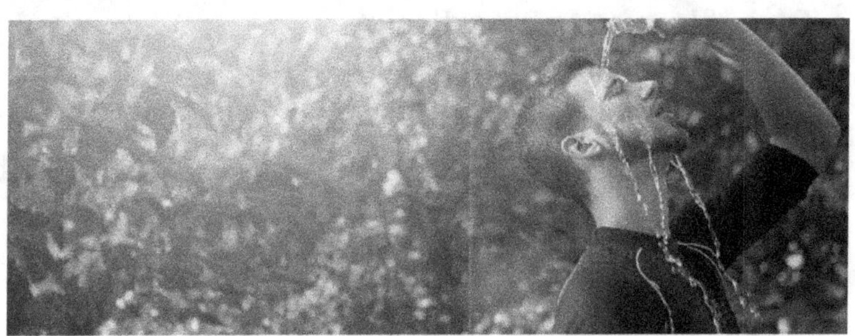

Ah, the delightful oasis in the health desert: water, the unsung hero of kidney care! In this chapter, we'll delve into the crystal-clear waters of comprehending the complex relationship between hydration and kidney health. Join the hydration party as we spill the beans on why hydration is so important and how to maintain proper fluid balance.

The Relationship between Hydration and Kidney Health

Consider your kidneys to be dedicated workers in a crowded factory, constantly filtering waste and maintaining your body's delicate fluid balance. Imagine this factory running efficiently with an abundant supply of water; this is the magic of hydration in kidney health.

1. Fluid Balance Maestros:**
- Your kidneys orchestrate hydration throughout the body.
- Adequate hydration ensures that your kidneys have enough fluid to efficiently filter waste and toxins from your bloodstream.

2. Toxin Flushers Extraordinaire:

Water acts as a cleansing agent for the kidneys, allowing them to operate optimally. - When you're properly hydrated, your kidneys can effectively remove toxins, excess salts, and urea from your body via urine.

3. Kidney Stone Prevention Patrol:

Dehydration can cause concentrated urine, which increases the risk of kidney stone formation. - Staying hydrated dilutes the minerals and salts in your urine, lowering the risk of kidney stones and maintaining your kidneys stone-free.

4. Blood Pressure Balancers:

Proper hydration is vital for managing blood pressure, which impacts kidney health.
When you're properly hydrated, your blood volume stays steady, which helps to maintain healthy blood pressure and reduces strain on your kidneys.

5. Maintaining Electrolyte Balance

Hydration helps balance electrolytes like salt, potassium, and chloride in the body. - When you're hydrated, electrolytes are properly dissolved in your bloodstream, which promotes smooth cellular function and general kidney health.

6. Optimal Urine Production:

Staying hydrated helps your kidneys generate enough urine to properly remove waste from your body.

Insufficient fluid consumption can result in concentrated urine, which raises the risk of urinary tract infections and other kidney problems.

In essence, water is the lifeblood of kidney health; it keeps your kidneys running smoothly, prevents kidney stones, controls blood pressure, and maintains proper urine production. So, raise a glass (of water) to your kidneys and keep them hydrated for a healthy and happy filtering system!

Tips to Maintain Adequate Fluid Balance

1. Water, the Elixir of Kidney Life: Make water your beverage of choice – it's the VIP ticket to kidney health. Aim for at least 8 cups (64 ounces) of water per day, with adjustments dependent on activity level and weather.

2. Fruit-Infused Hydration Fiesta: Enhance your hydration routine with fruit-infused water. Spice up your water with pieces of citrus, berries, or cucumber for a taste explosion that will keep you reaching for the water bottle.

3. The Herbal Symphony: Herbal teas are a calming addition to your hydration routine.
Choose caffeine-free herbal teas to provide diversity to your fluid consumption while keeping your kidneys in balance.

4. Juicy Dance Partners - Hydrating Fruits and Veggies: Enjoy hydrating fruits and vegetables. Water-rich alternatives such as watermelon, cucumber, and oranges satisfy your taste buds while also contributing to your overall fluid intake.

5. Instead of chugging, try the sip method. Sip water throughout the day rather than drinking it all at once; your kidneys like a continuous hydration tango.

As you begin your hydration journey, remember that water is more than simply a beverage; it's a love note to your kidneys. Maintain fluid equilibrium, dance with hydration, and allow your kidneys enjoy the aqueous embrace of wellness. Cheers to staying hydrated and keeping your kidneys happy and healthy!

CHAPTER 8

Expert Insights

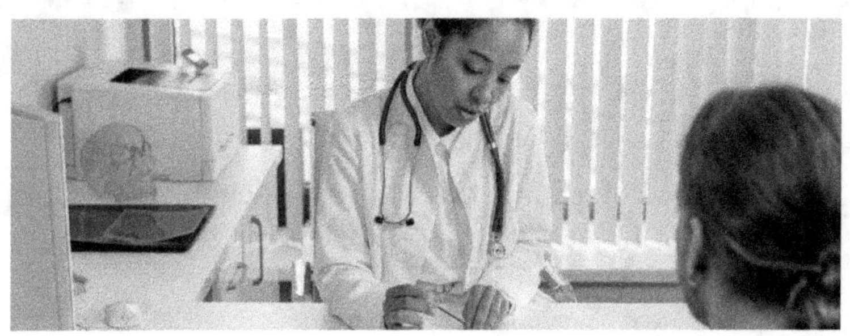

In this chapter, we're pleased to present you with a carefully curated collection of guidance and recommendations from specialists who traverse the complex landscape of kidney health.

Expert Insights from Nutritionists

1. Balancing Act – The Nutrient Symphony:

The importance of striking a balance between nutrients cannot be overemphasized.

Aim for a broad and colorful meal that includes a variety of fruits, vegetables, lean proteins, and whole grains to guarantee a full range of critical nutrients.

2. Portion Control Ballet:

The dance of portion control is a key theme in the expert playbook.

Pay attention to portion proportions to ensure you get a fulfilling meal without overloading your kidneys with nutrients.

3. Mindful Eating Meditation:

Practice mindful eating by savoring each bite, noticing hunger and fullness cues, and enjoying the sensory experience of your meals.

Insights From Healthcare Professionals

1. Individualized Nutrition Serenade:

Recognize that everyone's nutritional needs are different, and seeking individualized advice from a healthcare professional can help you improve your kidney health.

2. Hydration Harmonics:

Hydration is more than just drinking water; it's about maintaining a fluid balance that helps your kidneys work properly. Listen to your body's thirst cues and drink water throughout the day.

3. Collaborative Care Choreography:

Collaboration between nutritionists and healthcare practitioners is essential.

Encourage collaboration between your nutritionist and your healthcare team to ensure that you receive comprehensive care that includes both the dietary and medical elements of kidney health.

4. Lifestyle Rhythms for Kidney Wellness:

Incorporate regular exercise, stress management techniques, and adequate sleep into your daily routine to cultivate a balanced lifestyle that benefits your kidneys.

As you digest these expert advice, keep in mind that knowledge is your ally on the path to renal heath. Consult with healthcare specialists and nutritionists, accept individualized counsel, and allow expert insights to lead you down the path of optimal kidney health. May your journey be filled with insight, balance, and a symphony of wellness!

CONCLUSION

As we approach the final chapter of "Kidney Friendly Food List," let's take a moment to reflect on the wealth of knowledge we've discovered together - a journey that goes beyond dietary recommendations to encompass a holistic approach to kidney wellbeing. The symphony of insights, expert advice, and practical solutions has been crafted to help you achieve optimal kidney health.

Our journey began with comprehending the complexities of kidney health, delving into the principles of nutrition, and navigating the world of renal-friendly food options. We deciphered labels, discovered hidden causes, and even looked at the lifestyle elements that work in tandem with your kidneys. This symphony of information serves as a compass, guiding you to a life full of vitality.

We highlighted the significance of personalized care, mindful eating, and the collaborative choreography of lifestyle factors. Consider those recommendations as more than just words on paper, but as a transforming roadmap to improving your well-being.

Starting along the path to kidney-friendly living is more than simply a dedication to your physical health; it's a celebration of life's tastes. Each meal, every mindful bite, and every deliberate decision you make contribute to a healthy, kidney-friendly lifestyle. Remember that the goal of this journey is to learn how to nourish your body and enrich your life, not to restrict it.

As you finish this book, consider the next steps in your personal journey to kidney heath. You are prepared to enjoy the symphony of life, armed with knowledge, backed up by expert insights, and motivated by a desire to improve your health. May every decision you make, every meal you prepare, and every lifestyle change you make demonstrate your dedication to good kidney health.

As you venture out into the world beyond these pages, may your kidneys dance to the beat of well-being and each day be a melody of health and joy. Until we meet again on our journey to vibrant life, here's to nourishing kidneys, enriching lives, and embracing a dynamic future!

<u>My Little Request</u>

Thank You For Reading This Book!
I really appreciate all of your feedback and
I love to hear what you have to say.

I need your input to make the next version of this
book and my future books better.

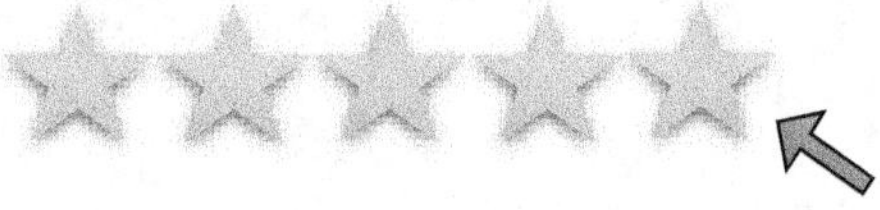

Please take two minutes now to leave a helpful 5-star
review on
Amazon letting me know what you thought of the book:
Thanks so much!
Bell Quintana

Attribution

All images used in this book were downloaded from *pixabay.com* and *pexels.com*.